Diagnosed with Diabetes!! Now What?

Smallest Book with Everything you need to know.

By
Dr. Shahriar Mostafa
MBBS, MPH

Notes

This book is not a prescription from doctor. Do not change, increase, start or skip any ongoing treatment without consulting your doctor.

Every effort has been made to make this book as complete and as accurate as possible. However, there may be mistakes both typographical and in content. Therefore, this text should be used only as a general guide and not as the ultimate source of information. Furthermore, this manual contains information on writing and publishing only up to the printing date.

Please visit the following Facebook page and hit like.
https://business.facebook.com/smallestbookonT1DM
I will send you every update / edition of this book (eBook only) completely free. You can also send an email to dr.shahriar@doctor.com . I will email you every update / edition of this book (eBook only) completely free.

Feel free to Email any question, suggestion or mistake to dr.shahriar@doctor.com I will answer your questions.

Without your review I can't reach others. I request you to write a review if you like or dislike this book. I will mention your review in future editions of this book. If you think this book may help a diabetic (your friends or family) please share the link of the book.

About Author

Dr. Shahriar Mostafa earned his MBBS degree in 2009. Then completed his Master's degree in Public Health in 2013. He has been working in a Medical College Hospital for last 7 years. He wants to write simple, easy to read and small patient education books to reach a larger audience.

Other Bestseller Books by Dr. Shahriar

Pregnancy & Diabetes: Smallest Book with Everything You Need to Know

http://www.amazon.co.uk/gp/product/B01CEDAH08

This book gives you a complete picture on GDM (Gestational Diabetes mellitus). It also gives information on pregnancy with type 1 or type 2 diabetes. If you are a pregnant mother with or without diabetes this book gives all the information you need to protect you and your baby from the complications of GDM or other types of Diabetes.

Type 1 diabetes: Smallest Book with Everything You Need to Know.

https://www.amazon.co.uk/dp/B01AQOJ21C

You can finish this book in just 1 hour. In just 1 hour you will have all important information on Type one diabetes. This book will give the confidence, hope and information to live a normal happy life with Type One Diabetes.

Type 2 diabetes: Smallest Book with Everything You Need to Know

https://www.amazon.com/dp/B01FUGZASK

As soon as you learn that you have Type 2 Diabetes you become terrified. What happens in Type 2 Diabetes? What to do to cure it? How to control it? What's causing it? Why did it happen to me? Thousand and thousand questions pop up in your mind. You become confused, afraid and angry. This book will answer all your questions.

Contents

Introduction

You were living your life to the full. Working hard and playing harder. Ignoring symptoms like fatigue, weight loss and increased frequency of urine. Then bam! Out of the blue you started feeling very sick. You consult with your doctor, he run some tests and you are diagnosed with diabetes!

Now what!

Should you leave all the things you love to do? Stop eating deserts. Adopt a life of Saints! Should you get panicked and think that's it, this is the end of the road! Well, it's not like that. Diabetes is a common disease. More than 350 million people in this world have diabetes. It's easy to control. It does not stop you living life to the fullest. You just have to keep it controlled.

Before we start the journey to know and control your diabetes here is a little about me. I have completed my MBBS from medical school 7 years back. Then did masters on public health. I have been treating people by working in a medical college hospital for last 7 years. I have written small and easy to read patient education books on diseases, especially on diabetes.

This is a small book. The purpose of this book is to provide you with all the latest information on diabetes. You can find all information on diabetes from internet, books and journals. But there is an ocean of information. Form this ocean of information finding what you really need is time consuming. And time is the most valuable thing of our life.

Because I have kept this book small, you can read this and save a lot of time. I have tried to keep the book as simple as possible and fun to read. You do not have to read this book from page one to the end. You can start anywhere and slowly finish it. Use the table of contents to find the topic of your interest and start from there. I sincerely hope that this book helps you living a normal, happy and fulfilling life, with diabetes.

Because diabetes is easy to control.

Now let's begin.

Chapter One: What is Diabetes.

Diabetes is a chronic disease, that means if you are diagnosed with diabetes it will stay with you all your life. But don't be alarmed. When properly controlled diabetes does not keep you away from anything life has to offer.

We call a patient Diabetic when he/ she has excessive glucose in blood. This condition of excessive and abnormally high glucose in blood is called Hyperglycemia. Persistent or continuous hyperglycemia is called diabetes. You must be thinking " From Where all this sugar is coming from!" Main source of sugar or blood glucose is the food we eat. The food we eat contains many substances. After eating, food is broken down into a simple form that our body can use. When food is broken into a simple form we get three major substances. Glucose or Sugar from Carbohydrate (rice, pasta, bread etc.). Fat from oil, butter etc. Protein from meat, milk egg etc.

For diabetes the carbohydrate or sugar part is important.

Carbohydrate starts its transformation from our mouth to stomach and intestine. Inside our gut food is mashed. Mixed with enzymes and acid and broken down into simple sugar or glucose. Glucose is the fuel used by our body to do everything we do and keep us alive. From our Gut glucose is absorbed to blood. Blood carries and delivers this glucose to every cell of our body. But glucose can't get inside every cell straight from the blood. For glucose to get inside our cells we need insulin. Insulin works as a key for glucose to get inside the cells of our body.

In our body, we have an organ called pancreas. Pancreas makes insulin. For any reason If pancreas could not make insulin. Or if your cells do not unlock its doors with insulin (insulin resistance).

glucose stays in the blood. This increased glucose level in blood or hyperglycemia is the condition we call Diabetes.

Diabetes is categorized in three major types. These types are based on functioning conditions of pancreas, its ability to produce insulin and time of onset of the disease. Let's get idea on all the types of diabetes

Type 1 diabetes
This type occurs mostly in children and young adults. Previously this type was called "juvenile onset diabetes Mellitus", it's also called insulin dependent diabetes Mellitus. "5-10 percent of all diagnosed cases of diabetes are type 1 Diabetes. Type 1 accounts for almost all the cases in children under age 10. Seventy-five percent of all cases of type 1 diabetes are in individuals under 18 years of age."

The environment around us has a vast number of microorganism. Every second microorganism such as bacteria, virus, fungus etc. enters our body. These bugs can make us sick. To prevent this our body has a natural defense mechanism. There are soldier cells such as Tcell & Bcells to fight against bacteria, virus, and cancer. In type 1 diabetes our body's defense mechanism malfunction. Solder cells of our body thinks cells of pancreas is harmful for us. These confused soldier cells attack and destroy insulin-making cells of the pancreas. With damage, pancreas can't make insulin anymore. Without insulin glucose can't get inside the cells. So glucose stays in blood and blood glucose level increases abnormally. This condition where pancreas can't make insulin anymore is called type one diabetes.

By definition, absolute deficiency or little production of insulin by pancreatic beta cells leading to hyperglycemia (high level of glucose in the blood) is called type one diabetes.

Type 2 diabetes

Type 2 develops over a long period of time (years). People with type 2 diabetes make insulin, but their cells don't use it as well as they should. One reason insulin may not work well is having excess body fat. The more body fat you have, the less likely it is that your insulin will work well. This condition is called insulin resistance. In insulin resistance, insulin becomes increasingly ineffective at managing the blood glucose levels. To correct this blood glucose level pancreas makes more insulin to try to get glucose into the cells. But eventually pancreas can't keep up, and glucose builds up in your blood causing diabetes.

"In adults 20 and older, more than one in every 10 people suffers from type 2 diabetes, and in seniors (65 and older), that figure rises to more than one in four. The International Diabetes Federation (IDF) reports that as of 2013 there were more than 387 million people living with diabetes. The World Health Organization (WHO) estimates that 90 percent of people around the world who suffer from diabetes suffer from type 2 diabetes."

Gestational diabetes or diabetes of pregnancy
Gestational diabetes is a specific type of diabetes which occurs during pregnancy. High blood glucose during the late phase of pregnancy (after 22 weeks) with no previous history of diabetes is called Gestational Diabetes. High blood glucose in an early phase of pregnancy (before 22 weeks) is not gestational diabetes. most likely its previously undetected type 2 diabetes. All pregnant women show some level of insulin resistance during late phase of pregnancy (after 22 weeks). But it does not reach too high level to be called diabetes.

Worldwide 3 to 5 % pregnant mothers develop GDM during the course of pregnancy. According to CDC, GDM occurs 1 in every 20 pregnancies. The alarming thing is the chance of getting GDM is increasing.

During pregnancy, our body makes more hormones. Extra hormones are needed to support the pregnancy and the growing baby. This high levels of pregnancy hormones can cause your blood glucose to rise. Changes during pregnancy also causes Insulin resistance. Insulin resistance means insulin cannot work properly to transfer glucose from the blood to cells. Insulin resistance also increases your body's need for insulin. If your pancreas can't make enough insulin glucose can't enter your cells. Glucose stays in blood and causes hyperglycemia or high level of glucose in blood.

This rise in blood glucose causes gestational diabetes.

Common Symptoms of all types of diabetes are;
Increased thirst - when blood glucose level is high. Our body tries to dilute the high blood glucose with water. To meet this increased water demand, body signals our thirst center. So thirst increases.

Increased frequency of urination- In diabetes frequency of urination increases. Diabetic patients have high blood glucose. To lower this blood glucose, body tries to flush out the extra glucose through urine. That's why increased frequency of urination occurs. Diabetic patients may pass urine for more than 20 times a day.

Increased volume of urine - in hyperglycemia or high blood glucose. The body tries to remove all excessive glucose through urine. So the volume of urine increases up to 3 liters or more.

Other common symptoms are;
Pain in abdomen.
Loss of appetite.
Nausea and vomiting.

Type 1 diabetes may cause dehydration, unconsciousness, recurrent episodes of urinary & genital tract infections

Type 2 diabetes develops over a long period of time (years). So the symptoms develop gradually. Symptoms of type 2 diabetes is almost same as type 1 diabetes, such as Increased thirst, Increased frequency of urination, Increased volume of urine.
Weight loss is a major sign of type 2 diabetes. If you are losing weight, even after taking enough food, you should consult your doctor to rule out type 2 diabetes.
Without any obvious cause excessive tiredness or fatigue is another symptom of type 2 diabetes.
Other symptoms of type 2 diabetes include;

Loss of appetite.
Nausea and vomiting.
Blurring of vision.
Mood change.
Irritability.

Gestational diabetes is usually diagnosed when routine lab tests are done for pregnancy. It does not show specific symptom or sign. During pregnancy some symptoms of diabetes is masked by symptoms of pregnancy (vomiting, nausea, tiredness and fatigue etc.)
There are some specific symptoms occur in gestational diabetes. These symptoms are called alarming symptoms. If you have any of the following symptoms (alarming symptoms) you must consult your doctor immediately.
Alarming symptoms of gestational diabetes;
A severe headache.
Your baby moves less or more than normal.
Severe swelling of face, fingers or feet.
Blurry vision with or without a headache.
Pain or burning when you urinate.
Fever.
Backache or period-like cramps that come and go.
Severe pain in any part of your body that does not go away.
Any spotting of red blood from your vagina (the birth canal).
Blister or sore in your vaginal area.
Smelly, thick or yellow mucous from your vagina.

Diabetes has a genetic predisposition which means you have an abnormal gene from your parents for diabetes. But this genetic defect also needs a trigger event or risk factor to cause disease. Some of the risk factors are modifiable. You can avoid modifiable risk factors to prevent or delay diabetes. Following are the risk factors of diabetes.

Risk factors of type 1 diabetes;

Many factors are responsible causing type one diabetes. To develop type 1 diabetes a person has to have;
A specific genetic defect in chromosome 6.
A trigger event such as;
A Viral infection (with Coxsackie B Virus Enterovirus, German measles (rubella), Mumps or Rotavirus) or Exposure to an antigen such as Cow's' milk.

When a mother has type one diabetes the child has 3 percent chance of getting type one diabetes. If the father has type one diabetes the child has 6 percent chance of getting it. But if both parents have type one diabetes the child has a 30 percent chance of getting type one diabetes.

Risk factors of type 2 diabetes:

Age – being over the age of 40 (over 25 for south Asian people) is a risk factor of type 2. This may be because people tend to gain weight and exercise less as they get older. However, despite increasing age being a risk factor for type 2 diabetes, over recent years' younger people from all ethnic groups have been developing the condition. It's also becoming more common for children, in some cases as young as seven, to develop type 2 diabetes.

Genetics – having a close relative with diabetes (parent, brother or sister). A child who has a parents with type 2 diabetes has about a one in three chance of developing it

Weight – You're more likely to develop type 2 diabetes if you're overweight or obese (with a body mass index (BMI) of 30 or more. In particular, fat around your tummy (abdomen) increases your risk. This is because it releases chemicals that can upset the body's cardiovascular and metabolic systems. With diabetes obesity increases your risk of developing a number of serious conditions, including coronary heart disease, stroke and some types of cancer.

Ethnicity – being of south Asian, Chinese, African-Caribbean or black African origin (even if you were born in the UK, USA or any other country) increase your chance of getting type 2 diabetes. Type 2 diabetes is up to six times more common in south Asian communities than in the general UK population, and it's three times more common among people of African and African-Caribbean origin.
People of south Asian and African-Caribbean origin also have an increased risk of developing complications of diabetes, such as heart disease, at a younger age than the rest of the population

Other risks

Your risk of developing type 2 diabetes increases if your blood glucose level is higher than normal, but not yet high enough to be diagnosed as diabetes. This condition is called "pre-diabetes" – sometimes it's called impaired fasting glycaemia (IFG) or impaired glucose tolerance (IGT).
Pre-diabetes can progress to type 2 diabetes if you don't take preventative steps, such as making lifestyle changes. Lifestyle

changes include eating healthily, losing weight (if you're overweight) and taking plenty of regular exercise.

Women who have had gestational diabetes during pregnancy also have a greater risk of developing type 2 diabetes in later life.

Risk factors of gestational diabetes;

Ethnicity – People of south Asian, Chinese, African-Caribbean and black African are more likely to develop gestational diabetes during pregnancy.

Weight – same as type 2 diabetes You're more likely to develop gestational diabetes if you're overweight or obese (with a body mass index (BMI) of 30 or more.

Women who have had gestational diabetes during previous pregnancy also has a greater risk of developing gestational diabetes again when pregnant.

Chapter Five: Diagnosis of diabetes

Besides symptoms, some tests are done to confirm diabetes. Your doctor will decide which tests are needed. Some common tests for diabetes are;

Fasting blood glucose - Done after overnight fasting (No food or drinks for at least 8 hours). You have to give a small amount of blood early in the morning on an empty stomach. If the test result shows fasting blood glucose level equal or more than 126 mg/dL (7.0 mmol/L). It is a positive of diabetes.

2 hours after 75g glucose - In this test after overnight fasting (No food or drinks for at least 8 hours). On an empty stomach, you have to take 75g glucose dissolved in a glass of water. Then after 2 hours, a small amount of blood taken to measure the glucose level in blood. Blood glucose level equal or more than 200 mg/dL (11.1 mmol/L) two hours after 75g glucose. Is positive for Diabetes.

A random blood glucose level can be done anytime. A small amount of blood taken. Random blood glucose equal or more than 200 mg/dL (11.1 mmol/L) is positive for diabetes. It indicates that your doctor should do other tests to confirm diagnosis of Diabetes.

A test called Hemoglobin A1c is essential.
HbA1c measure glucose in red blood cells. It shows the average blood glucose level for 2 to 3 months. It is also useful for treatment & follow up of a patient with Diabetes. This test can be done anytime. Empty stomach or just after food. Food has no effect on this test result. HbA1C level more than 6.5% is positive for diabetes. But if you have anemia, sickle cell anemia or thalassemia the test result can be false positive.

The HbA1C test should be performed in a laboratory using a method that is NGSP certified and standardized to the DCCT assay.

Type 1 diabetes needs some additional lab tests. Your doctor may do other tests such as;

Autoimmune markers include islet cell autoantibodies. Autoantibodies to insulin, autoantibodies to GAD (GAD65). Autoantibodies to the tyrosine phosphatases IA-2 and IA-2b. Autoantibodies to zinc transporter 8 (ZnT8).

Diabetic patients frequently have other associated diseases such as thyroid dysfunction, Celiac disease, Pernicious anemia, Addison's disease etc. To check other diseases. And to screen out the complications of diabetes following tests are done.

Complete Blood Count with Peripheral Blood Film
Serum ACTH level
Thyroid function test – to rule out thyroid dysfunction.
Fasting lipid profile – for vascular damage, heart diastase.
Liver function test.
Renal function test – to prevent of diabetic kidney disease (Diabetic Nephropathy).
Electrocardiogram (ECG) etc.

Lab tests for Gestational Diabetes Mellitus.
GDM is usually diagnosed by lab investigation. As soon as you become pregnant your doctor will do some tests as routine investigation.
Pregnant women with risk factors will be screened for undiagnosed type 2 diabetes at first prenatal visit. Your doctor may do fasting blood glucose & blood glucose 2 hours after breakfast test.
Pregnant women without any history of diabetes is screened at 24-28 weeks for Gestational diabetes.

For the diagnosis of Gestational diabetes, any one of the following types of diagnostic test is done. According to American diabetic association, the strategy to diagnose GDM as follow

"One-Step" Strategy

75-g glucose is given orally after fasting overnight or 8 hours. Blood glucose measured of fasting and at 1 hour and 2 hours. This test is done at 24-28 weeks of pregnancy in women not previously diagnosed with any diabetes or GDM.

GDM diagnosis made if blood glucose values are more than:
Fasting: 92 mg/dL (5.1 mmol/L)
1 h: 180 mg/dL (10.0 mmol/L)
2 h: 153 mg/dL (8.5 mmol/L)

"Two-Step" Strategy

50-g glucose is given orally. There is no need for fasting before the test. Blood glucose is measured 1 hour after oral glucose. It's done at 24-28 weeks of pregnancy.
If blood glucose at 1 h after oral glucose is ≥140 mg/dL (7.8 mmol/L), proceed to 100-g oral glucose tolerance test, this test needs fasting overnight or 8 hours.

GDM diagnosis made when two or more blood glucose levels meet or exceed:
Fasting: 95 mg/dL or 105 mg/dL (5.3/5.8)
1 hour: 180 mg/dL or 190 mg/dL (10.0/10.6)
2 hours: 155 mg/dL or 165 mg/dL (8.6/9.2)
3 hours: 140 mg/dL or 145 mg/dL (7.8/8.0)

Following tests are also done if you have Gestational diabetes. Ultrasound exams, which use sound waves to make images that show your baby's growth, approximate weight, genetic abnormalities if present and an expected delivery date. Ultrasound exams are completely safe for the baby.
A nonstress test, which uses a monitor placed on your abdomen to check whether your baby's heart rate increases as it should when your baby is active.

Chapter Six: Monitoring Blood Sugar at Home.

Monitoring blood glucose level in blood is important, especially for Type one diabetes. Getting pricked with Lancet or syringe 3 to 4 times every day is a painful process. But there is no better working alternative yet. You cannot guess the blood glucose level without a test. Only if the blood glucose level is low a patient can feel it, but even then he can't feel how low it is.

For Type one diabetes you should check the blood glucose level at least 3 times every day. Before every meal.
Once every week, check blood glucose one hour after meal. And once in every two weeks check blood glucose in the middle of a night.

Lab test result for blood glucose is almost same using glucometer at home. Glucometer test from the finger blood may vary only 10% of a lab test.

You must maintain a log with date, time, condition (empty stomach or after food) and blood glucose level. There are now apps available in iOS, android, and windows to easily maintain diabetes log.

Steps to check blood sugar at home?

Start the task of home blood glucose monitoring with making the meter ready. Insert the strip in meter. Wash your hand, you may clean the finger with rubbing alcohol or use soap and water. Prick finger to get 1 drop of blood. Give the blood on the strip. In few seconds, the meter will display current blood glucose level.
Do finger prick on the side of the finger where pain sensation is low. If available, use low pain lancet. It will reduce pain. Use alternate

finger every time. If blood does not come after finger prick by the Lancet, a gentle squeeze of the finger will help.

Carefully store glucometer strips. Only 2-hour exposure of strips to air will damage the strip. Blood glucose level from finger prick is better than blood from other sites (heel, ear lobe etc.)

Apps for record keeping of diabetes?

Monitoring and keeping the record of your Diabetes is easy now. There are many apps for iPhone, iPad, Android and Windows. To give you an initial idea of these I have reviewed two apps. You can use these apps or find one of your choice.

Diabetes: M

Designed for smartphones and tablets this application is intended to help diabetics to manage better their diabetes and keep it under control. Users can log their values in this diary and keep the records with them all the time. The application tracks almost all aspects of the diabetes treatment and provides detailed reports, charts, and statistics to share via the email with the supervising physician. It provides various tools to the diabetics, so they can find the trends in blood glucose levels and allows users to calculate normal and prolonged insulin boluses using it's highly effective, top-notch bolus calculator.

"Diabetes: M" can analyze the values from the imported data from various glucometers and insulin pumps via the exported files from their respective diabetes management software systems.

Supports Android Wear smartwatches. The app is available in Android play store and iTunes store.

mySugr Diabetes Logbook

mySugr Logbook app is a charming diabetes tracker for blood glucose, bolus, basal, food, carbs, meds, pills, weight, a1c and more. It makes your diary useful in everyday life with playful elements and immediate feedback through your diabetes monster! Get motivated and involved in your diabetes therapy, today!

— No. 1 diabetes logbook app in 6 countries

— Most popular diabetes logbook app in the world based on five-star reviews and ratings

— Winner of Germany's "Focus Diabetes" 'Best Apps for People with Diabetes' award

Our motto: We make diabetes suck less!

FEATURES/ADD-ONS:

• Designed for type 1 & type 2 diabetes
• Quick and easy logging (meals, meds, BG's, and more)
• Personalized logging screen (add, remove, and reorder fields)
• Estimated HbA1c - so there are no nastier surprises
• CGM data integration via CSV import (only available in German and English speaking countries)
• Daily, weekly, monthly analysis (and more)
• Exciting challenges for personal therapy goals

You can visit the iTunes store or google play store, there are a lot of apps for diabetes. You can download those apps and decide which app works for you.

You can modify your lifestyle to control diabetes and prevent complications. Lifestyle modification for healthy living is a major part of treatment of diabetes. For Type 1 diabetes lifestyle modification reduces the chance of complication. You can modify your lifestyle to manage diabetes without medicines. The goal of lifestyle modification is to Keep your blood glucose, blood pressure and cholesterol at target levels.

Regularly test your blood glucose level. For type one diabetes its 3 times daily before meals.
See your doctor for all your recommended screening tests.
Take your prescribed medicine regularly.
Quit smoking.
Exercise at least 30 min every alternate day.
Follow a diet plan. Consult a dietitian for specific diet plan for you.
Limit alcohol intake.
Maintain ideal weight.

With diabetes specifically for type 2 diabetes you'll need to look after your health very carefully for the rest of your life. After being diagnosed, or if you're at risk of developing diabetes, the first step is to look at your diet and lifestyle, and make any necessary changes.
Three major areas that you'll need to look closely at are your:
Diet
Weight
Level of physical activity
By eating healthily, losing weight (if you're overweight) and exercising regularly, you may be able to keep your blood glucose in a safe and healthy level without the need for other types of treatment or drugs.

Diet

Increasing the amount of fiber in your diet and reduce your fat intake, particularly saturated fat. A good diet plan can help prevent diabetes, as well as manage the condition if you already have it. You should;

Increase your consumption of high-fiber foods, such as wholegrain bread and cereals, beans and lentils, and fruit and vegetables.

Choose foods that are low in fat – replace butter, ghee and coconut oil with low-fat spreads and vegetable oil.

Choose skimmed and semi-skimmed milk, and low-fat yoghurts.

Eat fish and lean meat rather than fatty or processed meat, such as sausages and burgers

Grill, bake, poach or steam food instead of frying or roasting it

Avoid high-fat foods, such as mayonnaise, chips, crisps, pasties, poppadums' and samosas.

Eat fruit, unsalted nuts and low-fat yoghurts as snacks instead of cakes, biscuits, Bombay mix or crisps.

Weight

If you're overweight or obese (body mass index (BMI) of 30 or over is called obese), you should lose weight. By gradually reducing your calorie intake and becoming more physically active you can lose weight. Losing 5-10% of your overall body weight over the course of a year is a realistic initial target. You should aim to continue to lose weight until you've achieved and maintained a BMI within the healthy range, which is:

BMI 18.5-24.9kg/m² for the general population
BMI 18.5-22.9kg/m² for people of south Asian or Chinese origin ('south Asian' means Bangladesh, Bhutan, India, Indian-Caribbean, Maldives, Nepal, Pakistan and Sri Lanka)

If you have a BMI of 30kg/m² or more (27.5kg/m² or more for people of south Asian or Chinese origin), you need a structured weight loss program, which should form part of an intensive lifestyle change program. To achieve changes in your diet, you should consult a dietician or a similar healthcare professional for a personal assessment and tailored advice about diet and physical activity.

In case of gestational diabetes, you will gain weight. Gradual increasing weight is good for you. The amount of weight gain depends on your weight before pregnancy, your height and physical condition. Your doctor or dietitian will advise you the specific amount of weight you need. As a general rule;
Women who were underweight before pregnancy should gain 28 to 40 pounds
Women who were normal weight before pregnancy should gain 25 to 35 pounds
Women who were overweight before pregnancy should gain 15 to 25 pounds
Women who were obese before pregnancy should gain 11 to 20 pounds

Physical activity

Being physically active is very important in preventing or managing diabetes.
For adults who are 19-64 years of age, the physical activity guidelines are:

150 minutes (2 hours and 30 minutes) of "moderate-intensity" aerobic activity – such as cycling or fast walking – a week, which can be taken in sessions of 10 minutes or more, and muscle-strengthening activities on two or more days a week that work all major muscle groups (legs, hips, back, tummy (abdomen), chest, shoulders and arms)

An alternative recommendation is to do a minimum of:
75 minutes of "vigorous-intensity" aerobic activity, such as running or a game of tennis every week, and muscle-strengthening activities

on two or more days a week that work all major muscle groups (legs, hips, back, abdomen, chest, shoulders and arms)

In cases where the above activity levels are unrealistic, even small increases in physical activity will be beneficial to your health and act as a basis for future improvements.

Reduce the amount of time spent watching television or sitting in front of a computer. Going for a daily walk – for example, during your lunch break – is a good way of introducing regular physical activity into your schedule. If you're overweight or obese, you may need to be more physically active to help you lose weight and maintain weight loss. Your doctor, diabetes care team or dietician can give you more information and advice about losing weight and becoming more physically active.

For gestational diabetes physical activity is good for both mother and the baby. Exercise will help you use blood glucose. But before exercise or any physical activity talk to your doctor and health care team. They will tell you what exercise is safe for you. One of the best exercises for pregnant women is walking. Try to walk or exercise at least once a day. Do more if you can. Your goal is to walk twenty minutes after each meal. Walking after a meal helps lower your blood glucose. If your BMI was more than 27 before you became pregnant, you may be advised to take moderate exercise for at least 150 minutes (2 hours and 30 minutes) a week. But remember never start any physical activity or exercise without consulting your doctor.

Pregnancy with Type 1 or Type2

If you are a known diabetic with type 1 or type 2, you need to follow some rules to reduce the risk of developing complications during pregnancy.

Plan your pregnancy – as there are many risk involving pregnancy with diabetes you must plan your pregnancy. Consult your doctor as you start planning for pregnancy.

Control your blood glucose – if your blood glucose level is high most of the time you should avoid pregnancy until you have a good control. Usually your doctor would do a blood test called HbA1c which shows overall blood glucose control in last 3 months.

Start Supplements – your doctor will prescribe vitamin supplement and folic acid tablet as soon as you plan for pregnancy. In early weeks of pregnancy Folic acid is essential to prevent neural tube defect in the baby.

Do not be too worried if you got pregnant without planning. Just visit your doctor immediately.

Chapter Eight: Medical Treatment of Diabetes

Please note that "This book is not to be used as prescription or doctor's advice. To change, add or remove any treatment you must consult with your doctor or healthcare team. Author of this book is not responsible if you change, add or stop any ongoing treatment".

To evaluate the treatment of diabetes we setup some goals.
Primary goal of diabetes treatment is to control your blood glucose level.
Target Fasting blood glucose level with treatment is 6mmol/l and 2 hours after meal 8 mmol/l.
Target HbA1c level is less than 7%.

Another role of treatment of diabetes is to prevent complications. For this
Target blood pressure is under 140 / 80
Target LDL level is below 100.
Target blood cholesterol less than 4 mmol/L
Tryglicaroid level below 1.7 mmol/L.

Treatment with Medicine: sometimes blood glucose is not controlled with lifestyle modification alone. For this some medicine are used to control diabetes.

Type 1

Treatment for type 1 diabetes depends on age, weight and physical condition of patient. In type 1 diabetes pancreas do not make insulin anymore so to treat type 1 Diabetic patients we need to give insulin as injection. Insulin is a protein, if given by mouth(orally) it gets digested in stomach. So insulin is given as injection. The injection is given under the skin. If we give insulin in vein or muscle, it works fast but works for a very short time. That's why insulin is given under skin so that it is absorbed slowly and work for a long time.

Patient can take insulin by insulin pen, insulin pump or insulin injection under the skin.

Type one diabetes does not respond to oral medicine. Most of the people with T1DM needs a long acting basal insulin and a mealtime short acting bolus insulin. Detail information about Insulin is in next chapter.

Type 2

There's no cure for diabetes yet, so treatment aims to keep your blood glucose levels as normal as possible, control your symptoms & prevent complications. Type 2 diabetes usually gets worse over time. Making lifestyle changes, such as adjusting your diet and exercise, may help you control your blood glucose levels at first. But they will not be enough in the long term.

You may eventually need to take medication to help control your blood glucose levels. Initially, this will usually be in the form of tablets, and can sometimes be a combination of more than one type of tablet. It may also include insulin or other medication that you inject.

The decision about which medications are best depends on many factors, including your blood sugar level and any other health problems you have. Your doctor might even combine drugs from different classes to help you control your blood sugar.

Gestational diabetes (GDM)

 Treatment of gestational diabetes focuses mainly on medical nutrition therapy, exercise, and glucose monitoring aiming for the target blood glucose. Most of the time GDM is controlled with lifestyle modification only. There is very little or no data on the long-term effect of oral diabetes medicine in pregnancy. So Insulin is the preferred agent for management of diabetes in pregnancy. The requirement of insulin changes rapidly throughout pregnancy. You will need dose adjustment frequently.

As a general rule to control gestational diabetes in the first trimester, there is often a decrease in total daily dose of insulin. In the second trimester, rapidly increasing insulin resistance requires a weekly or biweekly increase in insulin dose. Due to the complexity of insulin management in pregnancy, you should visit a specialized center, if this resource is available.

Following are brief descriptions on medicine that can be taken by mouth or orally to control diabetes.

Metformin - It is available as oral tablet or capsule. Generally, metformin is the first medication prescribed for type 2 diabetes. It works by improving the sensitivity of your body tissues to insulin so that your body uses insulin more effectively. It makes your cells more responsive to insulin. It also works by reducing the amount of glucose that your liver releases into your bloodstream. Metformin is recommended for adults with a high risk of developing type 2 diabetes, whose blood glucose is still increasing towards type 2 diabetes, despite making necessary lifestyle changes.

If you're overweight, it's also likely you'll be prescribed metformin. Unlike some other medicines used to treat type 2 diabetes, metformin doesn't cause additional weight gain.
Nausea and loose motion are possible side effects of metformin. These side effects usually go away as your body gets used to metformin. If metformin and lifestyles changes aren't enough to control your blood sugar level, other oral or injected medications can be added.

Sulfonylureas - Sulfonylureas increase the amount of insulin that's produced by your pancreas. Examples of medications in this class include glyburide, glipizide and glimepiride.
You may be prescribed sulfonylurea if you can't take metformin, or if you aren't overweight. Sometimes you may be prescribed sulfonylurea and metformin together if metformin doesn't control blood glucose on its own.

Sulphonylureas can increase the risk of hypoglycemia (low blood glucose), because they increase the amount of insulin in your body.

They can also sometimes cause side effects including weight gain, nausea and diarrhea.

Meglitinides - These medications work like sulfonylureas by stimulating the pancreas to secrete more insulin. They're faster acting, and the duration of their effect in the body is short. They have a risk of causing low blood sugar (hypoglycemia). Weight gain is a possibility with this class of medications.

Thiazolidinediones - Thiazolidinedione medicines (pioglitazone) make the body's tissues more sensitive to insulin so that more glucose is taken from your blood. They're usually used in combination with metformin or sulphonylureas, or both. This class of medications has been linked to weight gain and other more-serious side effects, such as an increased risk of heart failure and fractures. You shouldn't take pioglitazone if you have heart failure or a high risk of bone fracture. Because of these risks, these medications generally aren't a first-choice treatment.

Another thiazolidinedione, rosiglitazone, is withdrawn from use in 2010 due to an increased risk of cardiovascular disorders, including heart attack and heart failure.

DPP-4 inhibitors - These medications help reduce blood sugar levels, but tend to have a modest effect. They don't cause weight gain. Examples of these medications are sitagliptin, saxagliptin and linagliptin.

GLP-1 receptor agonists - These medications slow digestion and help lower blood sugar levels. Their use is often associated with some weight loss. Exenatide and liraglutide are examples of GLP-1 receptor agonists. Possible side effects include nausea and an increased risk of pancreatitis.

Gliptins work by preventing the breakdown of a naturally occurring hormone called GLP-1. GLP-1 helps the body produce insulin in response to high blood glucose levels. But GLP is rapidly broken down so it can't work for long time. Now by preventing this breakdown, the gliptins (linagliptin, saxagliptin, sitagliptin and vildagliptin) prevent high blood glucose levels, but don't result in episodes of hypoglycaemia.

You may be prescribed a gliptin if you're unable to take sulphonylureas or glitazones, or in combination with them. They're not associated with weight gain.

SGLT2 inhibitors - These are the newest diabetes drugs on the market. They work by preventing the kidneys from reabsorbing sugar into the blood. Instead, the sugar is excreted in the urine. Examples include canagliflozin and dapagliflozin. Side effects may include yeast infections and urinary tract infections, increased urination and hypotension.

Exenatide is a GLP-1 agonist, an injectable treatment that acts in a similar way to the natural hormone GLP-1 . It's injected twice a day and boosts insulin production when there are high blood glucose levels. GLP 1 agonist reduce blood glucose without the risk of hypoglycaemia.
It also leads to modest weight loss in many people who take it. It's mainly used in people on metformin plus sulphonylurea, who are obese. A once-weekly product has also been introduced.

Another GLP-1 agonist called liraglutide is a once-daily injection (Exenatide is given twice a day). Like Exenatide, liraglutide is mainly used for people on metformin plus sulphonylurea, who are obese, and in clinical trials it's been shown to cause modest weight loss.

Acarbose

Acarbose helps prevent your blood glucose level from increasing too much after you eat a meal. It slows down the rate at which your digestive system breaks carbohydrates down into glucose.

Acarbose isn't often used to treat type 2 diabetes because it usually causes side effects, such as bloating and loose motion However, it may be prescribed if you can't take other types of medicine for type 2 diabetes.

Nateglinide and repaglinide

Nateglinide and repaglinide stimulate the release of insulin by your pancreas. They're not commonly used, but may be an option if you have meals at irregular times. This is because their effects don't last very long, but they're effective when taken just before you eat. Nateglinide and repaglinide can cause side effects, such as weight gain and hypoglycaemia (low blood sugar).

If you have diabetes, your risk of developing heart disease, stroke and kidney disease is increased. To reduce risk of developing other serious health conditions, you may be advised to take other medicines, including:
Anti-hypertensive medicines to control high blood pressure
A statin, such as simvastatin or atorvastatin, to reduce high cholesterol
Low-dose aspirin to prevent stroke
An angiotensin-converting enzyme (ACE) inhibitor, such as enalapril, lisinopril or ramipril, if you have the early signs of diabetic kidney disease

Since its discovery in 1921. Insulin has become the most prescribed drug in history.
As a drug Insulin is made from animals (cow, pig etc.) or Bacteria genetically engineered to make insulin same as human insulin.
Some manufactured insulin is modified to work better. Those modified insulins are called an insulin analog.

Types of Insulin

There are many types of insulin.
Rapid Acting Insulin as the name implies, this type of insulin works within 15 min of injection and works up to 4 hours.
Short-acting insulin or regular insulin starts working in 30 minutes. It continues work up to 6 hours.
Intermediate-acting Insulin - NPH gets into blood in 2 hours. And works up to 18 hours.
Long-acting insulin reaches blood in 3 or 4 hours after injection. And works up to 24 hours.
There is mixed insulin containing rapid acting insulin analog and medium or long acting insulin. Given before meals. They start to work 2 hours after injection.

The objective of injectable insulin is to duplicate the secretion of insulin by normal pancreas. Normal insulin secretion from pancreas has two parts:

Basal insulin - usually from a normal functioning pancreas, a small amount of insulin called the basal secretion of insulin circulates in the blood at all times. This can be duplicated in a patient with Diabetes by taking long-acting insulin. The other way of getting small amount of insulin continuously is with an insulin pump.

Basal insulin deals with the glucose produced by your liver. If you skip a meal, your basal insulin alone should be able to keep your blood glucose levels stable.

Bolus insulin- normally the pancreas secretes a larger amount of insulin at the time of meals, called the bolus secretion. This amount is duplicated by taking rapid acting insulin just before the meal or regular insulin 30 minutes before meals.
While basal insulin influences your blood glucose levels in between meals, it's the bolus (fast-acting) insulin that deals with the carbohydrate contained in any food and drink you have.

Insulin is manufactured in strengths of 100 units per milliliter. Your doctor will determine the dose of insulin consisting of a basal dose and a bolus dose. Usually insulin dose is calculated by Patients weight in kilogram and multiplied by 0.3.

The first time a patient takes insulin, the dosage is based upon a calculated total daily dose. Your doctor will make this decision on dose,

Dose of Insulin

Doctors usually follow these steps to calculate insulin dose: Multiply the weight of the patient in kilograms by 0.3. (for example if a patients' weight is 40 kg, insulin needed (40 multiplied by 0.3) 12 unit per day. Divide the total daily dose into basal and bolus dose by simply dividing it in half. (for example if patient needs 12 units per day he should get 6-unit basal dose and 6-unit bolus dose.
The basal dose is taken once or sometimes split into two times a day, usually in the morning (two third of the full dose) and/or (remaining one third) at bedtime. It is best to divide the basal dose into a large number of units in the morning and a few units at bedtime.
Your doctor will decide how much insulin you need.

Bolus dose of insulin is calculated using three major factors.
The level of the blood glucose before a meal – if before meal blood glucose is high you need to add two unit of insulin with your regular dose. If the premeal blood glucose is lower than ideal, you need to decrease two unit of insulin from your regular dose.

The amount of carbohydrate in your meal – generally for every 15 grams of carbohydrate 1-unit insulin is added. But the amount of adjustment varies with different people at different ages.

Whether exercise has been or is about to be done - Exercise generally lowers the blood glucose. But sometime exercise may increase blood glucose. Try to maintain a blood glucose of about 150 mg/dl during exercise. Take glucose in the form of three to four glucose tablets if the blood glucose falls below 100 mg/dl. Take rapid-acting insulin and wait to exercise if the blood glucose is over 300 mg/dl. Take half the usual dose before a meal before exercise if the blood glucose is satisfactory. Try to exercise around the same time every day.

Insulin Storage

You have to know how to store insulin. Keep the insulin you are currently using at room temperature in a cool, dry place and away from direct light. Best to keep it under 30 C. Cold insulin injection is painful. If you keep regular use insulin in a fridge be sure to take out insulin from fridge 30 minutes before using it. Keep it at room temperature for 30 min before giving injection.

Store insulin for a long period at 4 to 6-degree temperature. Don't place insulin in, or close to, the freezer compartment.

Never heat insulin or keep it beside the source of heat (oven, TV, locked car, radiator etc.)

For travel use a special cold bag or use a flask.

Check the expiration date and color of insulin. If there is clamps or the color changed do not use it.

Don't use insulin if:

Clear insulin has turned cloudy or changed color.
The expiration date has been reached.
Insulin has been frozen solid or exposed to high temperatures.
Lumps or flakes can be seen inside the vial.
The vial has been opened for more than 28 days.

Where to inject insulin

Insulin is given just under the skin for longer effect. And most of the time it's self-administered. It's easy to give insulin injection in your belly, back and thighs. But remember not to give insulin at the same site regularly. Rotate the sites every time.

Steps to give an insulin injection?

For type one diabetes, insulin injection is the treatment. Your doctor will calculate how much insulin needed (Dose). Also, the doctor will tell you how many times insulins is needed and type of insulin needed. Never change the dose or schedule without consulting your doctor first.
Follow these steps to give an insulin injection
Wash your hand with soap and water.
Check the insulin bottle for expiration date.
Check the insulin bottle for clamps, color change. If there is clamps or color change do not give insulin from that vial.

Wipe the cap of insulin bottle with an alcohol pad.

Clean skin where you will get the injection with alcohol pad or soap and water.

Pinch skin and fat with thumb.

Push the needle into your skin: With your other hand, hold the syringe at a 45-degree angle. Make sure the needle is all the way into the skin.

Let go of the pinched tissue before you inject the insulin

Inject the insulin: Press the plunger with your thumb.

Use slow and steady push until the insulin is gone.

Wait 5 to 10 seconds.

Pull out the needle: Pull out the needle at the same angle you put it in. Press your injection site with cotton for a few seconds.

Use Insulin syringes only once. Throw away used needles and syringes in a hard container so that the needles cannot stick through. Close the container with a screw-on cap. Keep the container out of reach of children and pets.

How to decrease pain when giving insulin.

Inject insulin at room temperature. If insulin is stored in the fridge, remove it 30 minutes before you inject it. Cold insulin injection is painful.

Remove all air bubbles from the syringe before the injection.

If you clean your skin with an alcohol pad, wait until it has dried before you inject insulin.

Relax the muscles at injection site.

Avoid changing direction of the needle during insertion or removal.

Do not reuse disposable needles. Because needles get blunt and cause pain.

Try numbing the area of injection by use of an ice cube. Keep the ice cube pressed to skin for 2 minutes just before injection.

Always use a different site to give the injection.

Diabetes affect other systems such as heart, kidney and nervous system. That's why diabetes is a serious disease. You must control your blood glucose or control your diabetes. Diabetes has some immediate complication and some long term complications.

Short-term or immediate complications of diabetes include hypoglycemia, diabetic ketoacidosis and Hyperosmolar Hyperglycemic Nonketotic Syndrome or HHNS

DKA (Diabetic Ketoacidosis)

It is a dangerous short term complication of diabetes; it frequently occurs in Type one diabetes. In type one diabetes pancreas can't produce insulin. Without insulin, glucose can't enter & work in the cell. This extra Glucose accumulates in blood, causing hyperglycemia.
Glucose is the main source of energy of our body. To function our body needs energy or glucose. To meet this energy demand when glucose is unavailable, stored fat of the body starts to breakdown. Beside energy breakdown of fat leads to ketone production. With ketone in blood, blood becomes acidic and this condition is called diabetic ketoacidosis.

The cause of DKA includes Infection (Pneumonia or lung infection or Urine infection). Missed insulin injection, trauma, stroke or heart failure.

DKA is a medical emergency and must be treated at a hospital.

To prevent DKA you should never miss insulin injection. Monitor symptoms of DKA, you should be able to recognize symptoms of DKA.

Fruity Smell of acetone is a major sign of diabetic ketoacidosis. With rapid & shallow breathing pattern.

Sweating with cold, clammy skin.

Increased thirst.

Abdominal pain, Nausea & vomiting.

Confusion or coma. These are symptoms of DKA (Diabetic Keto Acidosis).

In DKA blood sugar is high, more than 250mg/dl (13.8 mmol/L).

To confirm DKA a home urine test can be done. Checking Ketone in urine is confirmatory test of Diabetic Keto Acidosis (DKA). You can check ketone easily at home using a home kit. Using home kit Ketone is measured easily by putting a ketone strip into a tube containing urine.

  If blood glucose is above 250 mg/dl (13.8 mmol/L). Check urine for ketone. To do the test, collect urine in a plastic cup and place a ketone strip in urine. The strip will change color. Compare the color with color chart and you get the result. There are four possible results, negative, low, medium or high.

High ketones with high blood glucose mean that there is a chance of getting DKA (Diabetic ketoacidosis).

DKA is a medical emergency, treatment can only be given at hospital / clinic. You should contact your doctor or diabetes health team immediately.

Hypoglycemia

Hypoglycemia or low blood glucose is another short-term complication of diabetes. It is a common but dangerous condition. The good thing is hypoglycemia shows certain symptoms. Which makes it easy to recognize. Hypoglycemia symptoms start to show as soon as blood glucose level becomes 75 mg/dl (4.1 mmol/L) or lower. Symptoms include Anxiety, Irritability, Numbness in the lips, fingers, and toes.

Most of the time accidentally taking insulin in high dose causes hypoglycemia. Another cause of hypoglycemia is taking the wrong type of insulin. Other causes are missed meal or small amount of food, too much physical exercise. Some drugs may lower blood glucose leading to hypoglycemia. Such drugs are Beta blockers for hypertension, Aspirin for a headache etc.

Mild hypoglycemia is treated with a small portion of food. You have to take carbohydrate or sugar containing drinks.

When the blood glucose level becomes 65mg/dl (3.6 mmol/L) or lower it's called moderate hypoglycemia. Symptoms include Rapid heartbeat. The sensation of hunger. Sweating and Whiteness or pallor of the skin. Moderate hypoglycemia needs 4 to 5 glucose tablets or oral glucose.   Recheck blood glucose after 20 minutes. If blood glucose level is still low take more glucose tablet or powder and recheck again.

When blood glucose level is less than 55 mg/dl (3.05 mmol/L) it's called severe hypoglycemia. Symptoms include Confusion and trouble concentrating, Convulsions, Dizziness, Fatigue, Feeling of warmth, headache, Reduced consciousness or coma, and Slurred speech. Severe hypoglycemia is a medical emergency. Patient needs to be taken to hospital as soon as possible. Use a glucagon injection if prescribed by your doctor and available. Glucagon is a hormone, and it's given in severe hypoglycemia to protect the body.

Glucagon comes in a package containing powder glucagon and water for injection in 2 vials. A syringe with needle is also available. Check the expiration date of glucagon injection.

First, take water from a vial with syringe. Inject the water in the powder containing bottle. Shake to mix powder glucagon with water. Take mixed drug using the syringe and inject into muscle. In hip or upper arm.

You and family members should learn the symptoms of hypoglycemia. And how to give glucagon injection. You need to have glucagon injection, glucose monitoring device and sugar tablet with you at all time.

There are some common things you can do in any type of hypoglycemia or low blood glucose. If the patient is conscious and can take food by mouth. He should be given 3 to 4 glucose tablets or 15 grams of glucose powder with half glass of water or you can give 15ml or three teaspoons of honey. Recheck blood glucose 20 minutes. If the blood glucose level is still low, you can give more glucose tablet or honey. Instead of glucose tablet (if unavailable). You can give sugar containing drinks such as Apple or orange juice.

HHNS

Hyperosmolar Hyperglycemic Nonketotic Syndrome(HHNS) is a serious condition most frequently seen in older persons. It is a short term complication of diabetes. HHNS can happen to people with either type 1 or type 2 diabetes that is not being controlled properly, but it occurs more often in people with type 2 diabetes. HHNS is usually brought on by something else, such as an illness or infection.

In HHNS, blood sugar levels rise, and your body try to get rid of the excess sugar by passing it into your urine. You make lots of urine at first, and you have to go to the bathroom more often. Later you may not have to go to the bathroom as often, and your urine becomes very dark. Also, you may be very thirsty. Even if you are not thirsty, you need to drink liquids. If you don't drink enough liquids at this point, you can get dehydrated.

If HHNS continues, the severe dehydration will lead to seizures, coma and eventually death.

HHNS may take days or even weeks to develop. Know the warning signs of HHNS.

Warning Signs of Hyperosmolar Hyperglycemic Nonketotic Syndrome are;

Blood sugar level over 600 mg/dl

Dry, parched mouth

Extreme thirst (although this may gradually disappear)

Warm, dry skin that does not sweat

High fever (over 101 degrees Fahrenheit, for example)

Sleepiness or confusion

Loss of vision

Hallucinations (seeing or hearing things that are not there)

Weakness on one side of the body

If you have any of these symptoms, call someone on your health care team.

To avoid hyperosmolar hyperglycemic nonketotic syndrome, you should keep close watch on your blood glucose level when you're sick (you should always pay attention to your blood glucose level, but pay special attention when you're sick).

Talk to your healthcare professional about having a sick-day plan to follow.

Immediate complication of GMD

Gestational diabetes has some specific Immediate complication. When you have gestational diabetes you have high blood glucose, your baby will also have high blood glucose. Baby's pancreas has to make extra insulin to control the high blood glucose it gets from you. As the baby's pancreas makes more insulin to lower the high blood glucose, just after birth the baby may develop sever Hypoglycemia (low blood glucose) it's a dangerous condition for the baby. hypoglycemia may even cause death if not treated immediately.

Long-term complications of diabetes develop gradually. Uncontrolled blood glucose for a long time affects Brain & nervous system, blood vessels, eyes and kidneys. They can eventually be disabling or even life-threatening. Some of the potential complications of diabetes include:
Heart and blood vessel disease. Diabetes dramatically increases the risk of various cardiovascular problems, including coronary artery disease with chest pain (angina), heart attack, stroke, narrowing of arteries (atherosclerosis) and high blood pressure.
Long term complications of diabetes.

Diabetic neuropathy (Nerve damage)

Excess sugar can injure the walls of the tiny blood vessels (capillaries) that nourish your nerves, especially in the legs. This can cause tingling, numbness, burning or pain that usually begins at the tips of the toes or fingers and gradually spreads upward. Poorly controlled blood sugar can eventually cause you to lose all sense of feeling in the affected limbs. Damage to the nerves that control digestion can cause problems with nausea, vomiting, diarrhea or constipation. For men, erectile dysfunction may be an issue
You should be screened by doctor for diabetic peripheral neuropathy (DPN) once every year.

Managing Diabetic neuropathy and its complications;
Diabetic neuropathy — is a common but serious complication of diabetes.

Specific treatments exist for many of the complications of diabetic neuropathy, including:

Urinary tract problems. Antispasmodic medications (anticholinergics), behavioral techniques such as timed urination, and devices such as pessaries. Pessaries are rings which can be inserted into the vagina to prevent urine leakage — may be helpful in treating loss of bladder control. A combination of therapies may be more effective.

Digestive problems. Gastroparesis is a condition occurring due to diabetic neuropathy, in which the stomach empties too slowly or not at all. You can usually prevent gastroparesis by eating smaller, more-frequent meals, reducing fiber and fat in the diet, and, for many people, eating soups and pureed foods. Diarrhea, constipation and nausea may be helped with dietary changes, probiotics and medications.

Low blood pressure on standing (orthostatic hypotension) another complication of Diabetic Neuropathy. This is often helped with simple lifestyle measures, such as avoiding alcohol, drinking plenty of water and standing up slowly. Your doctor may recommend an abdominal binder, a compression support for your abdomen, and compression stockings. Several medications, either alone or together, also may be used to treat orthostatic hypotension.

Diabetic Neuropathy may cause Sexual dysfunction. Sildenafil (Revatio, Viagra), tadalafil (Adcirca, Cialis) and vardenafil (Levitra, Staxyn) can improve sexual function in some men, but these medications aren't effective or safe for everyone. When medications don't work, many men turn to vacuum devices, or, if these fail, to penile implants. Women may be helped with vaginal lubricants.

For some people, these symptoms are mild; for others, diabetic neuropathy can be painful, disabling and even fatal. Work with your doctor to determine the best approach to managing your diabetic neuropathy complications.

To prevent diabetic neuropathy strictly keeping blood glucose at ideal level is the only option.

Diabetic Retinopathy

This is one of the major long term complication of type one diabetes. Diabetes damage the blood vessels of the retina (diabetic retinopathy), potentially leading to blindness. Diabetes also increases the risk of other serious vision conditions, such as cataracts and glaucoma.

To prevent diabetic retinopathy or eye disease, you must control blood glucose level. Optimize glucose control will reduce the risk or slow the progression of complication.

Diabetic Nephropathy (Kidney damage)

In Diabetic nephropathy, your kidneys slowly become nonfunctional. Uncontrolled blood glucose for a long time or in case of patients with long standing Diabetes causes kidney disease. The kidneys contain millions of tiny blood vessel clusters that filter waste from your blood. Diabetes damage this delicate filtering system of kidneys. Severe damage can lead to kidney failure or irreversible end-stage kidney disease, which often eventually requires dialysis or a kidney transplant.

To prevent diabetic kidney disease, you must control your blood glucose. Optimize glucose control will reduce the risk or slow the progression of diabetic kidney disease.

You have to control blood pressure. Keep the blood pressure close to a normal range such as 120 / 80 mmHg.
Control fat in the blood. Keep fat level (LDL or HDL) within normal range.
Treat urinary infection if you have a urinary infection.
For people with diabetic kidney disease, reducing the amount of protein in diet is essential.

Every year you should get your urine checked for urinary albumin and estimated glomerular filtration rate (eGFR)

Foot damage.

Nerve damage in the feet or poor blood flow to the feet increases the risk of various foot complications. Left untreated, cuts and blisters can become serious infections, which may heal poorly. Severe damage might require toe, foot or leg amputation.

Alzheimer's disease.

Diabetes may increase the risk of Alzheimer's disease. The poorer your blood sugar control, the greater the risk appears to be. The exact connection between these two conditions still remains unclear.

Skin diseases in diabetes

Many skin conditions are unique to diabetes because of the treatment and complications of the disease. The most common and important skin complications are:

Bruises - occur because insulin needles cut blood vessels.

Vitiligo - (loss of skin pigmentation) is part of the autoimmune aspect of type 1 diabetes and can't be prevented.

Necrobiosis lipoidica - which also affects people without diabetes, creates patches of reddish-brown skin on the shins or ankles, and the skin becomes thin and ulcerated. Females tend to have this condition more often than males. Steroid injections are used to treat this condition, and the areas eventually become depressed and brown.

Xanthelasma - which are small, yellow, flat areas called plaques on the eyelids, occur in type one diabetes even when cholesterol isn't elevated. Treatment may not be necessary.

Alopecia - or loss of hair, occurs in people with type 1 diabetes, but the cause is unknown.

Insulin hypertrophy - is the accumulation of fatty tissue where insulin is injected. This condition is prevented by changing the injection site regularly.

Insulin lipoatrophy - is the loss of fat where the insulin is injected. Although the cause is unknown, this condition is rarely seen now that human insulin has replaced beef and pork insulin in diabetes treatment.

Diabetic thick skin - is thicker than normal skin, occurs in people who have had diabetes for more than ten years.

Complications of GDM

The Long term complication of gestational diabetes is twofold. Both the baby and mother develop complication.

When you have GDM you have high blood glucose, your baby will also have high blood glucose. This extra glucose in baby's blood is converted and stored as fat. So the baby grows larger than normal. It's called macrosomia—macrosomia makes normal vaginal delivery difficult and more dangerous for you and your baby. There is increased chance of needing cesarean section operation to deliver the baby.

After birth, the baby may have breathing problems, a condition called respiratory distress syndrome. This condition occurs in babies born from a mother suffering from GDM.

The chance of the baby developing neonatal jaundice is increased if the mother has GDM.

In case of Mother Gestational diabetes may increase your chances of

Preeclampsia – it's a condition where blood pressure is high and loss of protein through urine occur.

The GDM causes the baby to increase in size which makes normal delivery impossible so a surgery called Cesarean section is done to deliver the baby.

Mothers with GDM become depressed leading to clinical depression.

In future, the chance of developing Type 2 diabetes increases with GDM.

Other diseases with Type One Diabetes?

Another specific complication of type 1 diabetes is Type 1 diabetes is frequently associated with other diseases. Malfunctioning defense mechanism which causes type one diabetes can also cause other diseases. Some autoimmune diseases associated with type one diabetes are thyroid disease, autoimmune gastritis, celiac disease, autoimmune hepatitis etc.

Thyroid gland – 7 to 30% of patients with type one diabetes has thyroid disease. 25% of children with type one diabetes have thyroid disease. As our body's defense malfunction and destroy the insulin-producing cells it also destroys cells of the thyroid gland. Leading to hypothyroidism (low thyroid hormone). Sometimes hyperthyroidism (high level of thyroid hormone).

Hypothyroidism with type one diabetes increases the risk of hypoglycemia (low blood glucose). Your doctor will screen, thyroid auto antibodies (lab test using blood). It is predictive of thyroid dysfunction.

Celiac diseases are more common with type one diabetes. In celiac disease cells of small intestine reacts to gluten. Celiac disease should be ruled out in symptomatic type one Diabetic patient. Symptoms of celiac disease are Abdominal pain, recurrent loose motion, weight loss, etc. If the child has celiac disease with type one diabetes his diet plan is different. Gluten free diet will keep celiac disease patients' symptom free. Gluten is found in wheat, barley etc.

Food is a major component in the treatment of type one diabetes. It is important to consult with a dietitian for a personalized diet plan. Bread, rice, potatoes, pasta & other starchy foods are the source of carbohydrate. Carbohydrate is broken down to simple sugar in our body. It gives us all the energy we need. But carbohydrate is also the main source of glucose in the blood. We should watch how much carbohydrate we take with each meal. 40 to 60 percent of calories of our diet should come from carbohydrate.

Meat, fish, eggs, beans are sources of protein. Protein is needed for repair and growth of our body. Proteins do not have a direct effect on blood glucose. Protein is the main component of hormones, enzymes and antibodies. 10 to 20 percent of calories of our diet should come from protein. As part of a mixed meal, protein will slow the absorption of carbohydrate. Which is good for you.

Milk & dairy foods have essential vitamins and minerals. These products also have an effect on blood glucose.

Fruit & vegetables They contain essential vitamins. For a healthy diet fruit and vegetables are essential.

Goals of Nutrition Therapy for Adults with Diabetes

Goal one- Get a healthy and nutritious meal. Your food choice will help you achieve your desired blood glucose level, ideal body weight, target blood pressure. Your food choice will help you to prevent complications of diabetes.

Goal two – maintain the pleasure of eating. With type one diabetes there is restriction on how much you eat. There is no restriction on what you eat. A good nutrition therapy will restore the pleasure of eating.

<u>Goal three</u> – a nutrition therapy will provide the individual with diabetes practical tools for day-to-day meal planning.

Tips on food.

It's best to consult with a dietitian to get your personalized diet plan. There are some common tips to help you with your diet.
Eat more whole grains, fruits, & veggies. Limit or avoid foods that are high in fat, sugar, and white flour.
Always use low-fat milk, cheese, yogurt and dairy products.
Use pulses such as peas, beans or lentils to replace or reduce meat.
Cut and remove visible fat from meat, from poultry product remove skin.
When cooking, try to drain excess fat from meat before adding spices.
Try to grill or baking instead frying. Learn low-fat cooking methods.
Eat carbohydrate that is slow to absorb with low glycemic Index.
Eat pasta, basmati or easy cook rice, grainy bread such as granary, pumpernickel, rye, new potatoes, sweet potato, yam porridge, oats and natural muesli. These foods have low glycemic index so blood glucose will be low.

For fat Choose unsaturated fats or oils, such as olive, rapeseed and sunflower oil. These fat will help you to lose weight. You can reach your target cholesterol level with low fat diet.
Use less butter, margarine and cheese.
Eat fish at least once every week.
Eat one potion of fruit such as 1 apple or banana or any other fruit you like every day.
Avoid sugary drinks or smoothies.
Do not take more than 6g of salt per day. Less salt reduces blood pressure and heart disease.

Do not take alcohol more than 3 units per day. Half a pint of lager, ale, bitter or cider has 1-1½ units. Do not take alcohol on an empty stomach.

Tips on carbohydrate.

Eat carbohydrate (rice, pasta, etc.) in large chunks. It takes time to breakdown large piece of carbohydrate inside our gut. So glucose is absorbed slowly and blood glucose rises slowly.
Eat carbohydrate with fat to slow down absorption.

For rapid rise of blood glucose (in case of hypoglycemia) drink fruit juice or any beverage with food.

Small snacks in between meals keep your blood glucose at a consistent level which is good for you.

Glycemic Index

The glycemic index is a system of giving a number to every carbohydrate-containing foods according to how much each food increases blood sugar. The glycemic index itself is not a diet plan, but one of various tools — such as calorie counting or carbohydrate counting — for guiding food choices.

Many popular commercial diets, diet books and diet websites are based on the glycemic index, including the Zone Diet, Sugar Busters and the Slow-Carb Diet. The purpose of a glycemic index (GI) diet is to eat carbohydrate-containing foods that are less likely to cause large increases in blood sugar levels. The diet is a means to lose weight and prevent chronic diseases related to obesity such as diabetes and cardiovascular disease.

You might choose to follow the GI diet because you:

Want to lose weight or maintain a healthy weight
Need help planning and eating healthier meals
Need help maintaining blood sugar levels as part of a diabetes treatment plan

The GI principle was first developed as a strategy for guiding food choices for people with diabetes. An international GI database is maintained by Sydney University Glycemic Index Research Services in Sydney, Australia. The database contains the results of studies conducted there and at other research facilities around the world.

A basic overview of carbohydrates, blood sugar and GI values is helpful for understanding glycemic index diets.

Carbohydrates

Carbohydrates, or carbs, are a type of nutrient in foods. The three basic forms are sugars, starches and fiber. When you eat or drink something with carbs, your body breaks down the sugars and starches into a type of sugar called glucose, the main source of energy for cells in your body. Fiber passes through your body undigested.

Two main hormones from your pancreas help regulate glucose in your bloodstream. The hormone insulin moves glucose from your blood into your cells. The hormone glucagon helps release glucose stored in your liver when your blood sugar (blood glucose) level is low. This process helps keep your body fueled and ensures a natural balance in blood glucose.

Different types of carbohydrates have properties that affect how quickly your body digests them and how quickly glucose enters your bloodstream.

Understanding GI values

There are various research methods for assigning a GI value to food. In general, the number is based on how much a food item raises blood glucose levels in healthy research participants compared with how much pure glucose raises their blood glucose. GI values are generally divided into three categories:

Low GI: 1 to 55
Medium GI: 56 to 69
High GI: 70 and higher

For example, raw carrots have a GI value of 35. This means that if you eat carrots in a quantity that supplies 1.8 ounces or 50g carbohydrate your blood glucose level will be 35 percent of the blood glucose level after eating 1.8 ounces (50 grams) of pure glucose. It's confusing, I know. But easy when you know that high GI value means more glucose and usually bad for you.
Comparing GI values can help us to make healthier food choices. For example, an English muffin made with white wheat flour has a GI value of 77. A whole-wheat English muffin has a GI value of 45.

Limitations of GI values

One limitation of GI values is that they don't inform the quantity you would eat of a particular food. For example, watermelon has a GI value of 80, which would put it in the category of food to avoid. But watermelon has relatively few digestible carbohydrates in a typical serving. In other words, you have to eat a lot of watermelon to consume the standard test level of 1.8 ounces (50 grams) of digestible carbohydrates.

A GI value tells us nothing about other nutritional information. For example, whole milk has a GI value of 31 and a GL value of 4 for a 1-cup (250-milliliter) serving. But because of its high fat content, whole milk is a poor choice for weight loss or weight control.

The published GI database is not an exhaustive list of foods, but a list of those foods that have been studied. Many healthy foods with low GI values are not in the database.

The GI value of any food item is affected by several factors, including how the food is prepared, how it is processed and what other foods are eaten at the same time.

Glycemic Load (GL)

Limitation of GI values is that they don't inform the quantity you would eat of a particular food.
To address this problem, researchers have developed the idea of glycemic load (GL), a numerical value that indicates the change in blood glucose levels when you eat a typical serving of the food. For example, a 4.2-ounce (120-gram) serving of watermelon has a GL value of 5, which would identify it as a healthy food choice. For comparison, a 2. 8-ounce (80-gram) serving of raw carrots has a GL value of 2.
Sydney University's table of GI values also includes GL values. The values are generally grouped in the following manner:
Low GL: 1 to 10
Medium GL: 11 to 19
High GL: 20 or more

Low GI Diet
A GI diet prescribes meals primarily of foods that have low values. Examples of foods with low, middle and high GI values include the following:
Low GI: Green vegetables, most fruits, raw carrots, kidney beans, chickpeas, lentils and bran breakfast cereals

<u>Medium GI</u>: Sweet corn, bananas, raw pineapple, raisins, oat breakfast cereals, and multigrain, oat bran or rye bread

<u>High</u>: White rice, white bread and potatoes
Commercial GI diets may describe foods as having slow carbs or fast carbs. In general, foods with a low GI value are digested and absorbed relatively slowly, and those with high values are absorbed quickly.

Commercial GI diets have varying recommendations for portion size, as well as protein and fat consumption.

Benefit of GI diet

Studies of the benefits of GI diets have produced mixed results.
<u>Weight loss</u>
In a 2013 review of 23 published clinical trials of low-GI or low-GL diets, researchers concluded that the diets were "as effective as other dietary alternatives in inducing weight loss." In four of the studies, low-GI or low-GL diets resulted in statistically significant improvements in weight loss when compared with other diets. Ten studies showed a slight improvement — but not a statistically significant improvement — in weight loss.
In another 2013 review, researchers analyzed clinical trials that compared two or more specialty diets to various dietary guidelines, including those published by the American Diabetes Association and the European Association for the Study of Diabetes. The results showed that low-carbohydrate diets and Mediterranean diets provided more weight-loss benefit than low-GI diets. (A Mediterranean diet includes olive oil, legumes, whole-grain cereals, fruit, vegetables, and modest amounts of meat and dairy products.)
A large trial published in 2010 followed 773 participants who had lost weight on a low-calorie diet. During the six months following this weight loss, people who ate a low-GI, high-protein diet were

more likely to stick with their diet plan and not regain the weight they had lost.

Blood glucose control
A treatment goal for people with diabetes is to keep after-eating and average blood glucose levels as close to nondiabetic levels as possible. This tight control helps prevent or slow the development of complications associated with the disease.
Some clinical studies have shown that a low-GI diet may help people with diabetes control blood glucose levels, although the observed effects may also be attributed to low-calorie, high-fiber content of the diets prescribed in the study.

Cholesterol
Reviews of trials measuring the impact of low-GI index diets on cholesterol have shown fairly consistent evidence that such diets may help lower total cholesterol, as well as low-density lipoproteins (the "bad" cholesterol) — especially when a low-GI diet is combined with an increase in dietary fiber.

Appetite control
One theory about the effect of a low-GI diet is appetite control. The thinking is that high-GI food causes a rapid increase in blood glucose, a rapid insulin response and a subsequent rapid return to feeling hungry. Low-GI foods would, in turn, delay feelings of hunger. Clinical investigations of this theory have produced mixed results.
Also, if a low-GI diet suppresses appetite, the long-term effect should be that such a diet would result over the long term in people choosing to eat less and better manage their weight. The long-term clinical research does not, however, demonstrate this effect.
The bottom line is in order for you to maintain your current weight, you need to burn as many calories as you consume. To lose weight, you need to burn more calories than you consume. Weight loss is best done with a combination of reducing calories in your diet and increasing your physical activity and exercise.

Selecting foods based on a glycemic index or glycemic load value may help you manage your weight because many foods that should be included in a well-balanced, low-fat, healthy diet with minimally processed foods — whole-grain products, fruits, vegetables and low-fat dairy products — have low GI values.

For some people, a commercial low-GI diet may provide needed direction to help them make better choices for a healthy diet plan. The researchers who maintain the GI database caution, however, that the "glycemic index should not be used in isolation" and that other nutritional factors — calories, fat, fiber, vitamins and other nutrients — should be considered.

Children with type one diabetes may develop some emotional issues. They tend to develop low self-esteem. The child feels as if he must be a bad person or have done something wrong to have been stuck with such a disease

The child develops the idea that diabetes makes you less handsome or pretty than your friends.
The child or you may blame himself for the disease.
You or your child may think diabetes damages your brain and feels inferior.
There is continuous fear of complication. The special diets, medication and blood glucose monitoring is emotionally demanding.

Emotional issues should be treated by counseling and support from family and friends. Professional counseling helps to gain self-esteem, reduce depression.

Celebrities with T1DM

Diabetes does not keep you away from success in your life. You need to believe that and explain it to your child. Following are some celebrities with diabetes, it shows if you control your diabetes there is no problem getting what you want for life.

" Halle Berry - Diabetes didn't stop her from appearing as the super-powered mutant Storm in the X-Men movies.
 Nick Jonas - This 14-year-old star of the pop rock band the Jonas Brothers was diagnosed with type 1 diabetes in 2007.

Adam Morrison - Diagnosed with type 1 diabetes at age 14, Adam worked hard and made it all the way to the NBA where he plays basketball for the Charlotte Bobcats.

Gary Hall - This Olympic athlete didn't let type 1 diabetes stop him from earning a gold medal in swimming.

Elliott Yamin - After being diagnosed with type 1 diabetes at age 16, he went on to become one of the top singers on American Idol in 2006.

Vanessa Williams - Not only was Vanessa the first African-American Miss America, she is also a diabetic.

Doug Burns - Mr. Universe doesn't let his type 1 diabetes stop him from being an award-winning bodybuilder.

Jackie Robinson - The first black baseball player in the major leagues had diabetes.

Anne Rice - The famous vampire novel writer is a diabetic.

George Lucas - The creator of the Star Wars saga is a very mild type 2 diabetic.

Chris Dudley - Before Adam Morrison, Chris Dudley played in the NBA with type 1 diabetes.

Bret Michaels - The lead singer of Poison was diagnosed with type 1 diabetes at age six.

Bill and John Davidson - The big bosses at Harley Davidson Motorcycles are diabetic.

Mikhail Gorbachev - The former leader of the Soviet Union is a diabetic.

Johnny Cash - The famous country musician was a diabetic.

Elvis Presley - The former king of rock 'n roll had diabetes.

Sharon Stone - Halle's Cat woman co-star also suffers from type 1 diabetes.

Thomas Edison - The inventor of the light bulb was a diabetic.

HG Wells - The famed science-fiction author had diabetes.

Nicole Johnson - 1999's Miss America has diabetes.

Kendall Simmons - Busting heads on offense for the Pittsburgh Steelers keeps this diabetic athlete busy."

The list of Successful people or celebrities is a long one. Here I have given a small fraction. These peoples show you that diabetes (when controlled) does not get in your way to success. These success stories will give your child confidence to deal with type one diabetes.

Maintaining a Quality Life with Type 2 Diabetes.

To have a quality life and maintain it with Type 2 Diabetes you have to control your blood glucose level, blood pressure and blood cholesterol level.
The keys to maintaining a high quality of life with Type 2 Diabetes Are
Regular measuring of blood glucose and knowing how to respond to high and low blood glucose.

Get regular examination (6 months or yearly) by your doctor or healthcare professional.

Learn how to count carbohydrate quantity in meals and adjust insulin dose accordingly.

Enjoying good food that's also nutritious.

Exercise regularly to keep your muscles in excellent shape This will help to keep your metabolism functioning well.

Get sufficient sleep at least 8 hours every day.

Avoiding blaming yourself when things don't go exactly as you planned.

Living with Type 2 Diabetes.

There are few things you can do to improve your life with Type 2 Diabetes.

Maintain a balance between control and freedom. Do not try to control every high blood glucose. It will stress you out. Focus on overall correction of blood glucose.

Anger with Type 2 Diabetes is a natural response. We become angry with all the limitations due to Type 2 Diabetes. Talk to your friend or family. Try to find out the specific cause of anger. Sometimes you should get some freedom from strict routine lifestyle.

Be aware that you should never blame yourself for the fact that you have diabetes. Type 2 Diabetes doesn't result from consuming too much sugar, failing to exercise sufficiently, or any other failure that you may imagine.

Don't overreact to any temporary loss of control or increased glucose level. Try to find the cause. Control of the blood glucose may be lost temporarily when you get sick with a virus or other problems. When it happens, move on and try to restore the control as soon as possible.

Recognize that depression can occur in patients with Type 2 Diabetes. If your sleep is disturbed, if you don't feel like eating, if your usual positive outlook changes to sadness and unhappiness, it may be the time to consult your doctor.

Type 1 diabetes, mainly occurs in children. It's difficult to explain the condition to your child. You have to teach him to live with the disease and have a positive attitude. Let the child take control of his diabetes, let him or her decided what should be eaten, how much play or exercise is good.

Appreciate achievements such as normal blood sugar, healthy eating.

Teach him to recognize the symptoms of complication.

You and your child must understand that it is not possible to control every high blood glucose. The true goal is to keep overall control of blood glucose level.
Diabetes does not have any effect on IQ or good looks.
By giving your child a positive attitude you can lead him to a successful life.
Explain to your child that many successful people have diabetes.

Caring for children with Type One Diabetes of all ages
Children with Type one diabetes have different reaction to diabetes at different age. Young children passively but not happily accept the insulin shots, whereas young adults want to take charge of their condition.

Infants up to 18 months

Most of the time diagnosis of Type One diabetes is missed in infants. Infants can't tell about their problems. You have to look for the symptoms like frequent diaper change due to increased urination. Persistent vomiting is also a sign of type one diabetes. Consult your doctor for a screening test of type one diabetes.

The infant up to 18 months of age with T1DM is completely under the care of his parent (usually the mother). He'll resist his shots and his glucose tests but you must clearly understand that they're essential. This is something you have to insist upon even though the child can't understand the reason.

It's best for the baby to prevent neurological symptoms, allow his blood glucose to be a little higher than normal. A blood glucose between 150 and 200 mg/dl (8.3 to 11.1 mmol/L) is a good target.

Toddlers between 18 months and 3 years

The toddler who is 18 months to 3 years old is at the stage of beginning to test his parents, establishing himself as a separate human being. He's starting to learn to control his environment (by toilet training, for example). With diabetes, he may refuse shots, refuse to eat enough and at the right time, and generally make it difficult for you to manage the disease. You have to set limits and be firm, know when to insist when the item is essential (like taking insulin) and when to give in so that the child can have some victories as well (like allowing the child a piece of birthday cake). Use of very short-acting insulin is helpful in toddlers because the child's eating habits tend to be irregular and you can give the insulin just as the child begins to eat.

Children between 3 and 6 years

The child between ages 3 and 6 is still home and tests your limitations even more than a toddler. But he can tell you when he has symptoms of hypoglycemia. At this age, the child is wondering what he did to deserve diabetes when all his friends don't have it. Get the child involved with food preparation so that he feels he plays a part in his care. As your child gets closer to 6 years old, think about enrolling him in a diabetes camp or a children's diabetes group. There he'll be surrounded by kids like him and will realize that everyone has similar concerns and limitations.

Don't try to teach your young child about the complications of diabetes yet. He doesn't possess the skills or knowledge to manage his disease and will simply be frightened.

Children between 6 and 12 years

As the child begins school between 6 and 12 years of age, he wants to know more. This is the time for you and the child to go to a diabetes education program and to sit down together with a dietitian to work out the best diet to promote continued growth and good diabetic control. It's also the time to hand over some of the control (don't give up control of the insulin just yet), especially because you're not at school to monitor the child all the time. Establish that the school has food that's healthy for your child and also has a program where knowledgeable people are available to help him in the event of hypoglycemia.

Teens between 13 and 15 years

When the child reaches age 13 to 15 and officially becomes a teenager, he's extremely curious and wants to know about everything, including his diabetes. Another trip together to a diabetes education program and the dietitian is essential. At this age, involving both parents in diabetes education and treatment is even better than just one parent.

This and the following stage may be a very difficult time in terms of trying to keep good glucose control because of the production of large amounts of growth hormone, which tends to raise blood glucose. Don't expect perfect blood glucose level.

Teens between 15 and 19

The stage of puberty, from age 15 to 19, with all the new and powerful hormones (especially the sex hormones) may prove to be the most difficult time of all to manage T1DM. All the problems of attraction to and being attractive for a significant other seem to get in the way.

Tips for Parents of T1DM.

Learn as much as you can on Diabetes. Use internet, medical handout and books.
Talk with your child. Give him/her courage. Teach him / her self-care for diabetes.
Make sure your child wears a medical identification product such as bracelet or pendant.

Communicate with school health team. Talk to school nurse. Give school an emergency contact address and Cell phone number. Provide all necessary items needed to maintain your child's health plan at school.

Chapter Fifteen: Future of Diabetes

In near future complete cure of type one diabetes will be available. There is extensive research ongoing to create an oral and intranasal insulin. Soon we will have oral or nasal spray insulin. The painful injection will not be needed anymore.

Stem cell is another latest treatment. Type one diabetes patient gets an infusion of stem cells which helps pancreas to regenerate and produce insulin.

Other drugs such as PDX1 are being developed. It's a protein. It will help to regenerate beta cells of the pancreas. To stop the destruction of beta cells, new drugs are being developed. The goal is to prevent T cells from killing beta cells of the pancreas.

This is an exciting time. All new drugs and treatment options are in human trail. In a few years' scientists hope to cure type one diabetes.

We now know that the problem in type 2 diabetes relates to high fat levels in the pancreas and the liver. When calorie intake is sharply decreased - either by a diet, or by weight loss surgery - the fat levels in these organs decrease and it has been shown that the function of the pancreas and liver returns to normal.

A single injection each week, which could help the body respond more appropriately to food, and at the same time would help with weight control. It is the future of type 2 diabetes treatment. This is what GLP-1 agonists do. These drugs, which mimic a naturally occurring gut hormone, that tell the body to produce more insulin and the brain to stop eating. These are already available, and a long-acting injection is well on its way.

Conclusion

Thank you for reading this book. I wish you a safe, healthy and fulfilling life with diabetes. If a single patient is helped through this book and information that is the biggest success of this book. The biggest success of me.

I humbly request you, please write a small review (1 or 2 lines) of this book. Share the link with your friends, family or coworkers, if you think this book can help with their diabetes.

You may visit the following Facebook page and hit like. I will send you every new update / edition of this book (eBook only, not printed) completely free.

https://business.facebook.com/smallestbookonT1DM

You can also send an email to dr.shahriar@doctor.com
I will email you every new update / edition of this book (eBook only, not printed) completely free. Feel free to Email any question, suggestion or mistake in the book to dr.shahriar@doctor.com I will answer your questions. Include your review and questions in future editions.

Thank you for your time.

***

www.ingramcontent.com/pod-product-compliance
Lightning Source LLC
Chambersburg PA
CBHW070330190526
45169CB00005B/1835